How Many Feet in the Bed?

Heather Spergel

Hand drawn illustrations by **Anita Martino**

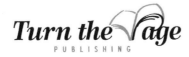
Turn the Page
PUBLISHING

Published by Turn the Page Publishing
PO Box 3179, Upper Montclair, NJ 07043

Copyright 2012 Heather Spergel

Distributed by
First Edition Design Publishing
www.firsteditiondesignpublishing.com
May 2012

Hand drawn artwork by Anita Martino
Design by Jeremy Rech

ISBN 978-1962287-000-4
LIBRARY OF CONGRESS CONTROL NUMBER 2012937344

Special thank you to my Granny (Gertie) for mysteriously and repeatedly waking me at 4 am to write (as I knocked heads with kids and cats desperately searching for a pen). For taking me seriously, I thank Julie and Roseann. To Anita, I am in awe of your beautifully drawn artwork. Thank you for jumping on the crazy bus with me in doing this project—I always knew you could do this! Family and friends— Love you! To my kids who inspire me daily, xo! H.S.

To my amazing family and friends, I am so grateful to have you along for the ride. Heather and Roseann, my partners in crime, words cannot express my gratitude; thank you for believing in me.
H.P. - I got this. —Anita

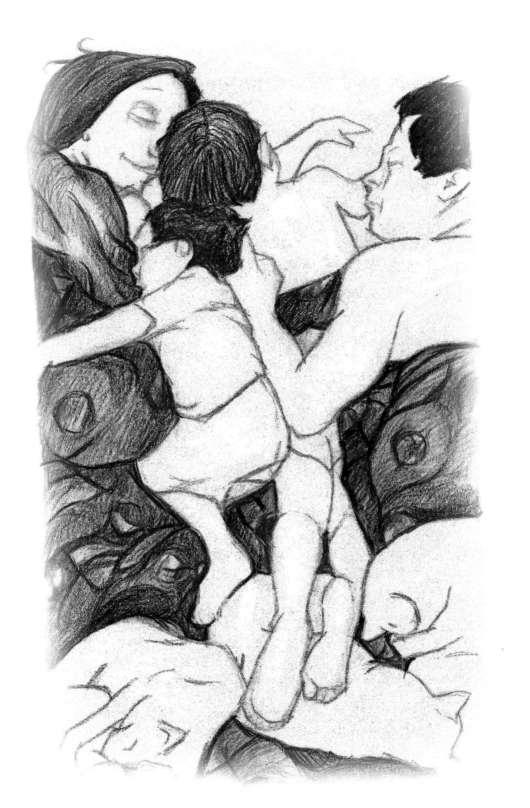

One bed
all alone

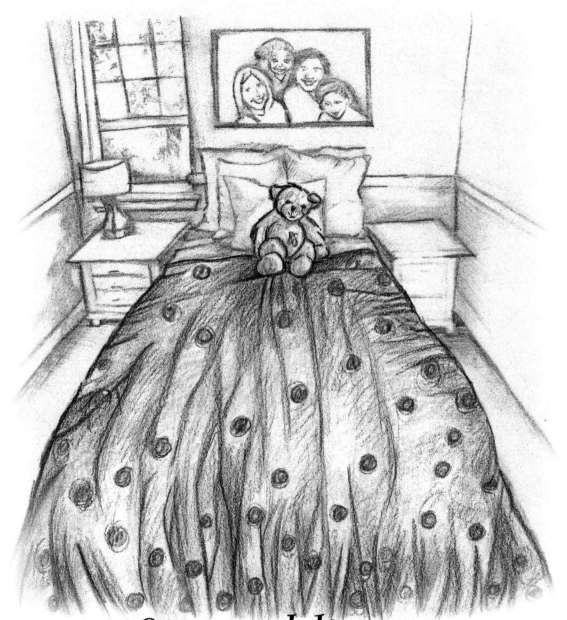

Sits and listens
to a happy home

2 Children too
excited for sleep

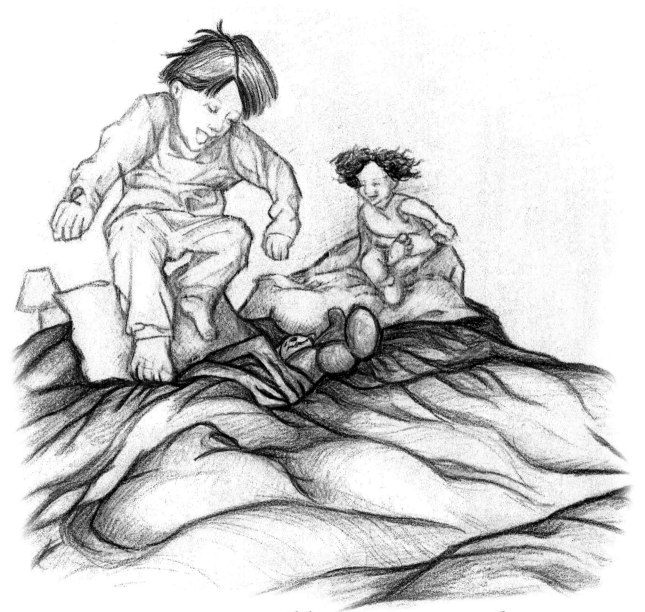

Jump all over and
dance and screech

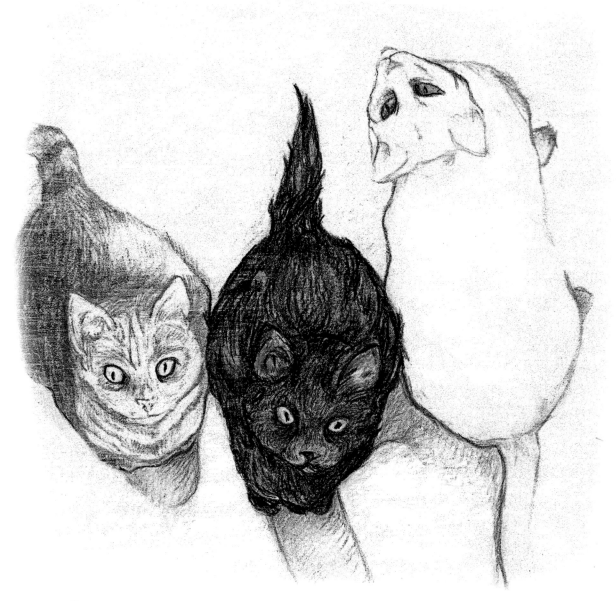

3 Kitties wanting some covers

Wonder when
the Fun might
be over

4 People
climb in close

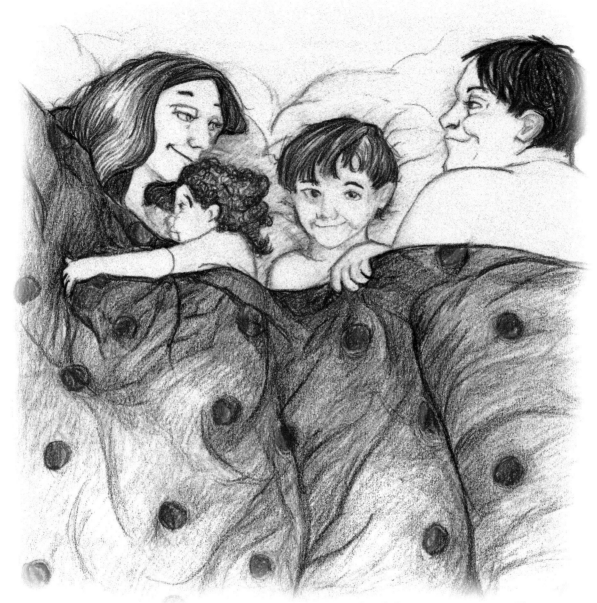

Everyone cuddles and
children nurse

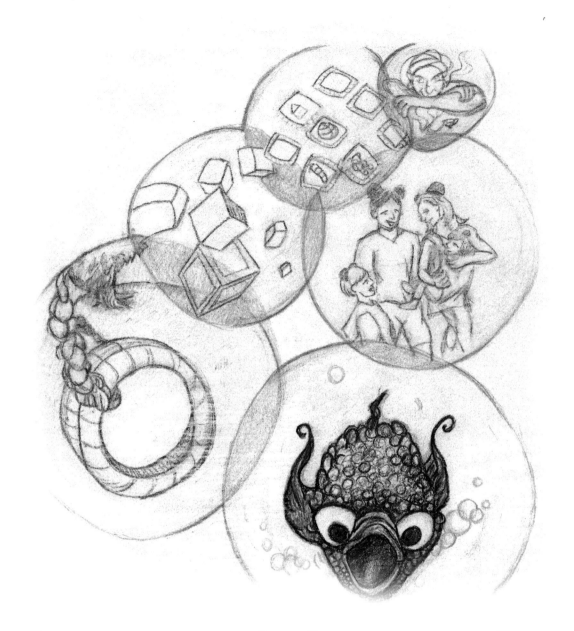

5 Dreams of Happy Wishes

Games

Toys

Trips

Parks

& Fishes

6 Sleepers
snooze away

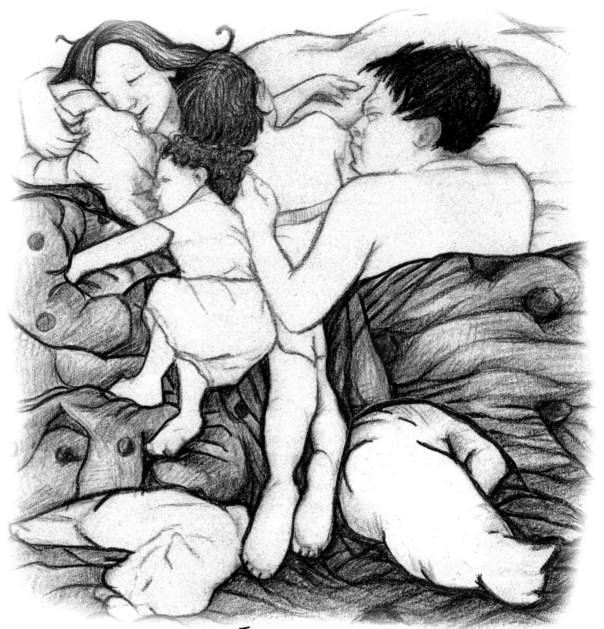

As night continues
its gentle play

7 Snuggle
and somehow
find room

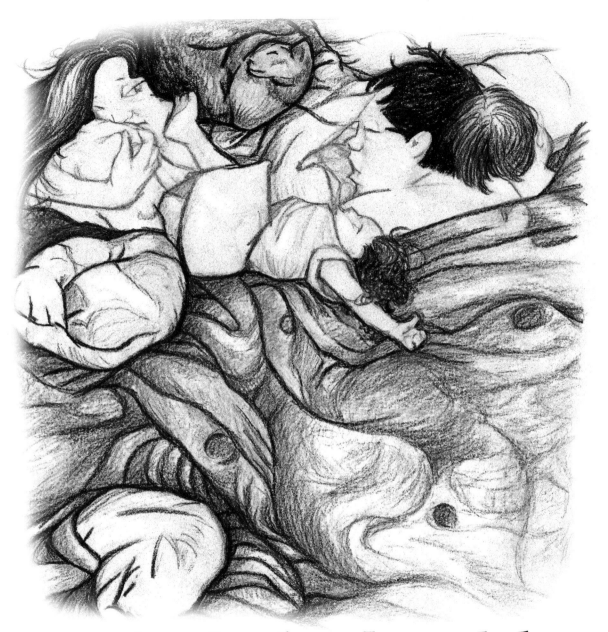

As the day breaks and the
sun peeks through

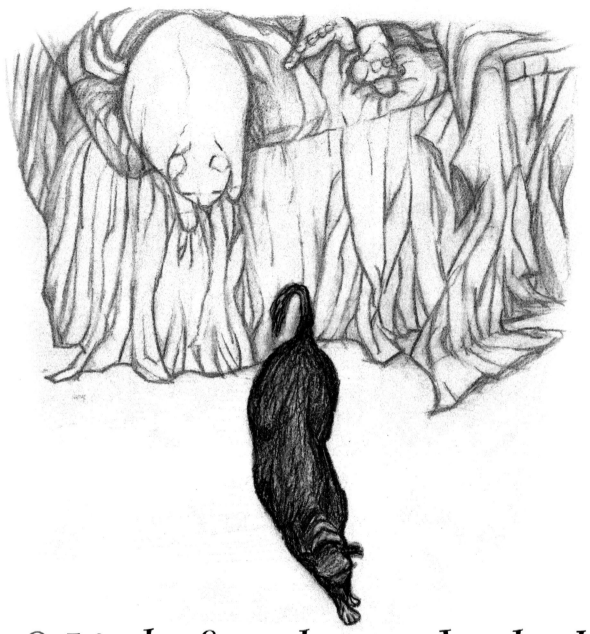

8 Little feet leave the bed

Hoping they will soon be fed

9 Hours
this sweet
group slept

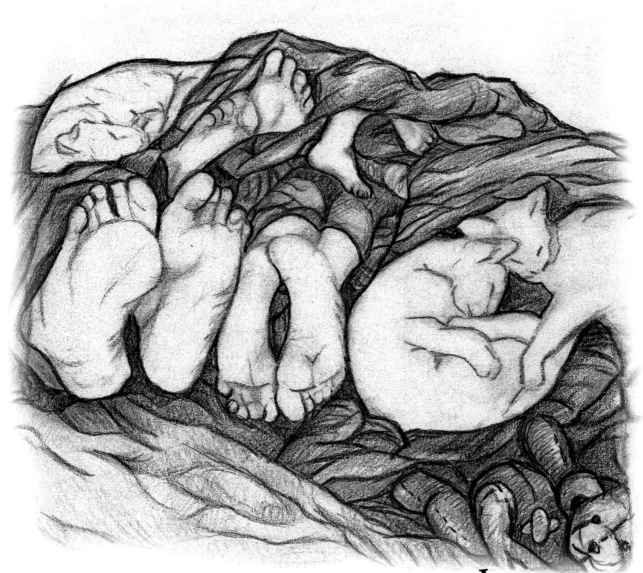

Feet intertwined
and comforts met

10 Minutes
cuddling as we
start our day

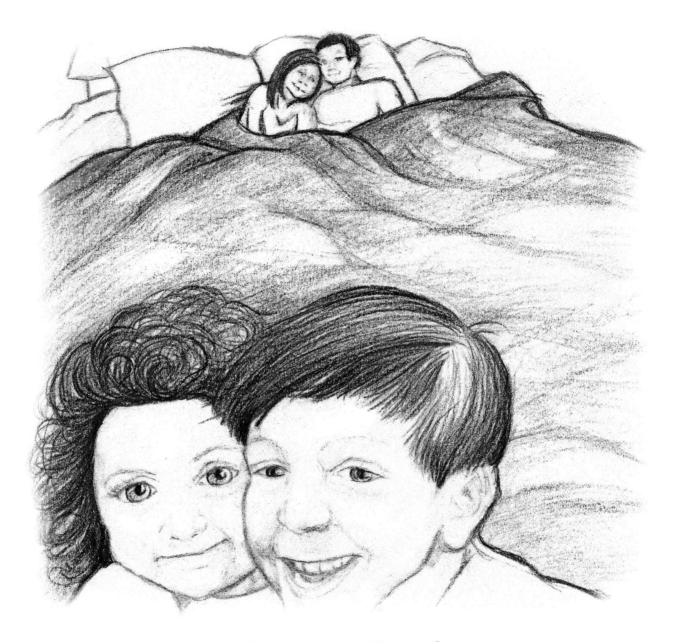

Snuggles and whispers
while kids run away

Good day,
sweet bed, we
say to you

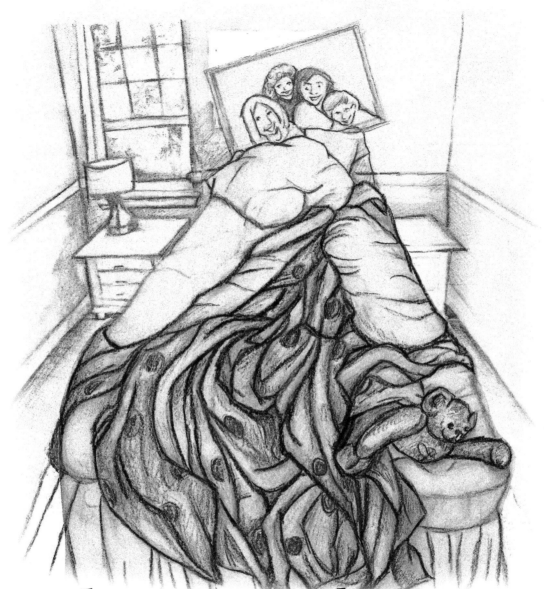

When we need our rest
we'll return to snooze.

Author's Note

As a bed sharing mom of two kids and way too many cats, our room sure is cramped. Laughing about it one night served as inspiration for this little book. One foot on my head, another pushing my legs sideways, a cat spooning me, and my husband falling off the bed—these are funny nights for us! I would not trade them for the world!

Cuddling and being close to one another is what works best for our family. Maybe this works well for you, or maybe some version of this works (less cats?). Or maybe it doesn't work for you at all. This book is not meant to be an instructional manual for how to sleep or how to raise your children. The book was written to share the humor in the parenting choices that we made as a family.

Whatever your bedtime looks like, laugh along with us as we count all the people and animals in our bed!

Activity with your child:
Search and find the teddy bears on the pages of the story.

How many do you see?

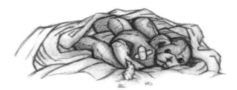

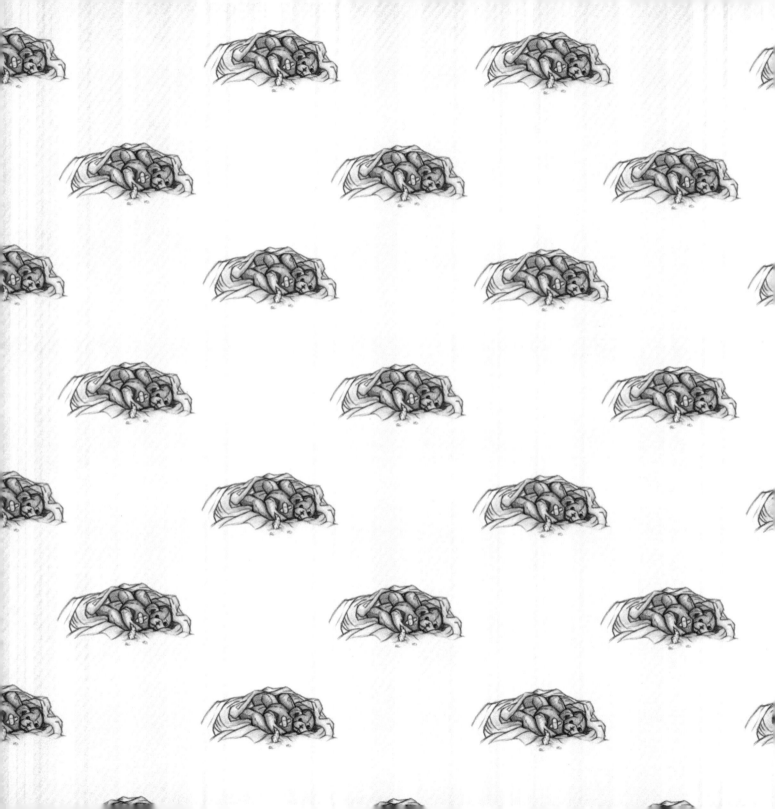

CPSIA information can be obtained
at www.ICGtesting.com
Printed in the USA
LVIC080954150512

281775LV00002B

9781622870004